The Anti-Histamine Diet Solution

Combat Allergies Naturally

By

Linda A. Ivey

Copyright © by Linda A. Ivey 2024.

GAIN ACCESS TO MORE BOOKS FROM ME

Table of Contents

Introducion to Histamine

Intolerance

Histamine intolerance is a condition that is garnering increasing attention as more people become aware of its impact on health and well-being. Understanding histamine intolerance involves delving into the intricate workings of our bodies' immune and digestive systems, as well as the role that histamine plays in these processes.

Histamine is a natural compound produced by the body and is involved in several essential functions, including regulating stomach acid production, neurotransmission, and immune response. It is released by specialized cells called mast cells and plays a crucial role in the body's defense against pathogens and foreign invaders.

However, for some individuals, the body's ability to properly metabolize histamine becomes impaired, leading to an excess buildup of this compound in the bloodstream. This accumulation can trigger a wide range of symptoms, collectively known as histamine intolerance.

The symptoms of histamine intolerance can vary widely from person to person and may include:

- Skin rashes, hives, or eczema
- Headaches or migraines
- Digestive issues such as abdominal pain, bloating, diarrhea, or constipation
- Nasal congestion, sneezing, or sinus issues
- Fatigue and brain fog
- Anxiety, irritability, or mood swings

It's essential to note that histamine intolerance is distinct from a histamine allergy, which involves a specific immune response to histamine or histamine-releasing foods. Histamine intolerance is more about the body's inability to break down and eliminate histamine efficiently, leading to an accumulation of the compound and subsequent symptoms.

Diagnosing histamine intolerance can be challenging, as there is no single definitive test for the condition. It often involves a process of exclusion, ruling out other potential causes of symptoms and tracking dietary and lifestyle factors that may exacerbate or alleviate symptoms.

One of the primary strategies for managing histamine intolerance is through dietary modification. Certain foods are naturally high in histamine or trigger the release of histamine in the body and may need to be limited or avoided by individuals with histamine intolerance.

Additionally, factors such as **stress, medications, alcohol consumption, and environmental allergens** can also influence histamine levels and exacerbate symptoms of intolerance.

In this book, we will explore the science behind histamine intolerance, the role of diet and lifestyle factors in managing symptoms, practical strategies for identifying and avoiding histamine triggers, and ways to support overall health and well-being in the presence of histamine intolerance.

By gaining a deeper understanding of histamine intolerance and implementing targeted interventions, individuals can take control of their health and enjoy improved quality of life. Whether you're newly diagnosed or have been managing histamine intolerance for years, this book aims to provide valuable insights and practical guidance to support you on your journey toward wellness.

Chapter 1

The Science Behind the Anti-Histamine Diet

- ## How Diet Affects Histamine Levels

The link between food and histamine levels is a complicated and intricate element of histamine intolerance and other diseases. Understanding how food choices affect histamine levels in the body is critical for those suffering from histamine intolerance.

Histamine is found in many foods, either as a natural component or as a result of microbial fermentation. Certain foods contain greater quantities of histamine, while others may increase histamine release or decrease the function of histamine-metabolizing enzymes. Consuming foods that raise histamine levels or interfere with histamine clearance might worsen symptoms and cause severe responses in histamine-sensitive people.

1. Foods With High Histamine Content: Histamine-rich foods include aged cheeses, cured meats, smoked salmon, sauerkraut, and fermented drinks such as wine, beer, and kombucha. These foods have higher amounts of histamine owing to the enzymatic breakdown of histidine, an amino acid found in protein-rich meals, during the fermentation or aging process. Consuming histamine-rich meals may lead to histamine buildup in the body, especially in those with poor histamine metabolism.

2. *Foods that release histamines:* In addition to histamine-rich meals, certain foods may cause mast cells or basophils to produce histamine, increasing histamine excess. Citrus fruits, tomatoes, strawberries, shellfish, and chocolate are common histamine-releasing foods. While these foods may not necessarily contain large quantities of histamine, they can cause the release of histamine in sensitive people, resulting in histamine intolerance.

3. *Histamine-Degrading Enzymes:* Histamine metabolism is principally controlled by two enzymes: diamine oxidase (DAO) and histamine N-methyltransferase. DAO breaks down ingested histamine in the digestive system, while HNMT metabolizes it inside cells and tissues. Certain dietary variables may affect the activity of these enzymes, either increasing or decreasing their function. Alcohol, black tea, and some medicines, such as nonsteroidal anti-inflammatory drugs (NSAIDs), may all suppress DAO function, reducing histamine clearance and increasing symptoms of histamine intolerance.

Individuals with histamine intolerance may reduce histamine exposure and symptoms by learning how nutrition influences histamine levels and metabolism. The anti-histamine diet focuses on eating fresh, unprocessed foods low in histamine and histamine-releasing substances while avoiding or restricting high-histamine foods and factors that interfere with histamine clearance. Adopting a personalized anti-histamine diet based on individual sensitivities and triggers may help people manage histamine intolerance successfully and enhance their overall quality of life.

- Foods High in Histamine

Here are some common categories of foods that are high in histamine:

1. *Fermented Foods*:

Fermentation is a process that involves the breakdown of sugars by bacteria and yeast. During fermentation, histamine levels can increase significantly. Foods such as aged cheeses (e.g., Parmesan, cheddar, blue cheese), sauerkraut, kimchi, yogurt, kefir, and sourdough bread are known to contain high levels of histamine. While fermented foods offer probiotic benefits for gut health, individuals with histamine intolerance may need to limit their consumption or choose alternatives.

2. *Cured and Aged Meats:*

Certain meats undergo curing, smoking, or aging processes that can elevate histamine levels. Examples include smoked or cured meats like bacon, sausage, salami, and ham. These products often contain added preservatives and flavorings, which can further increase histamine content. Opting for fresh, unprocessed meats or exploring plant-based protein sources can be beneficial for those with histamine sensitivity.

3. *Seafood:*

Fresh seafood is generally low in histamine, but histamine levels can increase as fish and shellfish age or undergo improper storage. Tuna, mackerel, sardines, anchovies, and shellfish like shrimp, crab, and lobster are prone to histamine accumulation if not handled and stored correctly. Individuals with histamine intolerance may find it helpful to consume freshly caught or flash-frozen seafood to minimize histamine exposure.

4. *Alcohol:*

Certain alcoholic beverages, particularly wine, beer, and champagne, contain histamine due to the fermentation process. Additionally, some alcoholic drinks may contain sulfites, which can trigger histamine release in sensitive individuals. Red wine, in particular, is notorious for its histamine content and is often associated with allergic reactions and headaches in susceptible individuals. Choosing low-histamine alcoholic alternatives or enjoying alcohol in moderation can help mitigate symptoms.

5. *Pickled and Fermented Vegetables:*

Pickled vegetables, such as pickles, olives, and relishes, can contain elevated levels of histamine due to the fermentation process. Similarly, condiments like soy sauce, vinegar, and mustard may also contribute to histamine load. While these foods can add flavor and variety to meals, individuals with histamine intolerance may need to exercise caution and moderation when consuming them.

6. *Citrus Fruits:*

While citrus fruits like oranges, lemons, and grapefruits are rich in vitamin C and other beneficial nutrients, they can also contain histamine-releasing compounds. Some individuals with histamine intolerance may find that consuming citrus fruits exacerbates their symptoms, particularly if they are sensitive to other histamine-rich foods. Monitoring individual responses to citrus fruits and moderating intake can help manage histamine-related reactions.

7. **Tomatoes and Tomato Products:** Tomatoes are another common trigger for individuals sensitive to histamine. While fresh tomatoes may be well-tolerated by some, processed tomato products like ketchup, tomato paste, and

pasta sauce can have higher histamine levels due to concentration and cooking processes. Individuals with histamine intolerance may opt for fresh tomatoes or homemade sauces prepared with fresh ingredients to minimize histamine exposure.

8. *Spinach, Eggplant, and Avocado:*

Certain vegetables and fruits contain naturally occurring histamine or histamine-releasing compounds that can contribute to symptoms in sensitive individuals. Spinach, eggplant, and avocado are examples of foods that some people with histamine intolerance may need to limit or avoid, especially if they experience adverse reactions after consumption.

Understanding the histamine content of foods and how they can influence histamine levels in the body is essential for individuals following an anti-histamine diet. By making informed dietary choices and prioritizing fresh, minimally processed foods, individuals with histamine intolerance can effectively manage symptoms and improve their overall quality of life.

- Histamine-Producing Bacteria and Fermented Foods

Fermented foods have been a part of global culinary traditions for millennia, revered for their robust flavors, rich textures, and possible health advantages. However, in the context of histamine intolerance, the complex connection between histamine-producing bacteria and fermented foods has significant relevance.

Fermentation is a natural process caused by the metabolic activity of microorganisms such as bacteria, yeast, and molds. These microbes degrade carbohydrates and sugars in meals, resulting in the synthesis of a variety of chemicals, including histamine. Certain bacteria have the enzymatic machinery required to convert histidine, an amino acid found in protein-rich meals, into histamine during fermentation.

Let's look further into the relationship between histamine-producing bacteria and certain widely ingested fermented foods.

1. *Cheese:* The world of cheese making is intriguing, with microbes playing an important part in flavor development and texture. Lactic acid bacteria like Lactobacillus and Streptococcus flourish in the cheese environment when it ripens. These bacteria produce decarboxylase enzymes, which aid in the conversion of histidine to histamine, adding to the particular flavors and qualities of aged cheeses. Gouda, Roquefort, and Camembert are just a few cheeses noted for their varied flavor profiles created by histamine-producing bacteria.

2. *Fermented veggies:* From sour sauerkraut to spicy kimchi, fermented veggies are appreciated for their high probiotic content and culinary variety. Lacto-fermentation occurs when naturally existing bacteria convert carbohydrates into lactic acid, resulting in an acidic environment that retains and improves the vegetable flavor. However, some kinds of bacteria engaged in fermentation may create histamine as a metabolic byproduct. While fermented veggies provide various health advantages, those who are sensitive to histamine may need to limit their intake to avoid negative responses.

3. *Yoghurt and Kefir:* Cultured dairy products, such as yogurt and kefir, are popular for their creamy texture and probiotic qualities. Lactic acid bacteria ferment milk, converting lactose into lactic acid, which gives it a tangy and somewhat sour flavor. While fermented dairy products provide helpful bacteria for gut health, some people may develop histamine-related symptoms as a result of the presence of histamine-producing bacteria in the fermentation culture. Shorter fermentation times or non-dairy alternatives may be good for persons with histamine sensitivity.

4. *Soy sauce,* a fundamental condiment in many Asian cuisines, is fermented to increase its savory umami flavor. Traditional soy sauce is made by fermenting

soybeans and wheat to produce a diverse palette of flavors and fragrances. However, the fermentation process might lead to the buildup of histamine, which can be problematic for those who are sensitive to it. Those suffering from histamine sensitivity may need to switch to low-sodium soy sauce or experiment with other condiments.

Understanding the relationship between histamine-producing bacteria and fermented foods is critical for those dealing with histamine sensitivity. While fermented foods have a variety of flavors and possible health advantages, they may be difficult for histamine-sensitive people to consume. Individuals may successfully manage histamine-related symptoms by implementing mindful consuming behaviors, experimenting with fermentation methods, and obtaining advice from healthcare specialists.

Chapter 2

Principles of the Anti-Histamine Diet

- Elimination and Rotation of High-Histamine Foods

Histamine intolerance presents a unique challenge in the realm of dietary management, requiring individuals to adopt strategic approaches to minimize histamine exposure while maintaining a balanced and nutritious diet. Two key strategies that form the cornerstone of managing histamine intolerance are the elimination and rotation of high-histamine foods.

1. Elimination of High-Histamine Foods:

a. Understanding Triggers:

- Identifying and eliminating foods high in histamine is the first crucial step. This involves recognizing common culprits such as aged cheeses, fermented products, certain seafood, and alcoholic beverages.

- Keeping a detailed food diary can aid in pinpointing specific triggers and understanding individual sensitivities.

b. Adopting a Low-Histamine Diet:

- Transitioning to a low-histamine diet involves avoiding or minimizing the intake of foods known to be rich in histamine. This includes processed and fermented foods, cured meats, and certain fruits and vegetables.

- Opting for fresh, unprocessed alternatives and selecting cooking methods that minimize histamine formation can be beneficial.

c. Reading Labels and Ingredients:

- Developing the habit of reading food labels becomes essential. Many processed foods contain hidden sources of histamine, such as preservatives, colorings, and flavor enhancers.

- Choosing whole, unprocessed foods and cooking from scratch whenever possible provides greater control over histamine intake.

d. Consulting Healthcare Professionals:

- Seeking guidance from healthcare professionals, such as dietitians or allergists specializing in histamine intolerance, can provide personalized advice. They may conduct tests to assess histamine levels or recommend elimination diets tailored to individual needs.

2. Rotation of High-Histamine Foods:

a. Introducing Variety:

- Rotation diets involve diversifying food choices to avoid consistently consuming high-histamine items. This approach prevents the accumulation of histamine over time.

- Incorporating a wide range of fruits, vegetables, proteins, and grains ensures a nutrient-rich diet while minimizing the risk of overwhelming histamine sensitivity.

b. **Timing and Frequency:**

- Rotating foods based on their histamine content requires paying attention to timing and frequency. For example, if a particular high-histamine food is well-tolerated in small quantities, it might be consumed occasionally rather than regularly.

- Monitoring symptoms and adjusting the rotation schedule based on individual responses is crucial for optimizing this strategy.

c. **Seasonal Eating:**

- Adapting the rotation approach to seasonal availability can be beneficial. Embracing fresh, locally sourced produce in season allows for a dynamic and varied diet.

- Seasonal eating also aligns with the philosophy of consuming foods at their peak nutritional value.

d. **Balancing Macronutrients:**

- In addition to rotating high-histamine foods, maintaining a well-balanced diet with an appropriate distribution of macronutrients (proteins, fats, and carbohydrates) contributes to overall health and supports the body's ability to manage histamine.

The elimination and rotation of high-histamine foods are not one-size-fits-all solutions but rather personalized strategies that require observation, experimentation, and adaptation. Finding the right balance often involves a trial-and-error process, with individuals gradually discovering their unique tolerance levels and dietary preferences.

Embracing these strategies empowers individuals with histamine intolerance to take an active role in managing their symptoms and improving their overall quality of life. By combining these dietary approaches with lifestyle modifications and seeking guidance from healthcare professionals, individuals can cultivate a sustainable and nourishing relationship with food while navigating the complexities of histamine intolerance.

- ## Importance of Fresh and Whole Foods

In the realm of histamine intolerance, dietary choices play a pivotal role in managing symptoms and promoting overall well-being. Embracing fresh and whole foods forms the cornerstone of an effective strategy for individuals navigating histamine sensitivity. Here's why:

1. Minimizing Histamine Exposure:

- Fresh foods, particularly fruits, vegetables, and lean proteins, are inherently low in histamine compared to their processed or aged counterparts.

- By prioritizing fresh and minimally processed options, individuals reduce their overall histamine intake, mitigating the risk of symptom flare-ups and allergic reactions.

2. Preservation of Nutrient Integrity:

- Fresh foods are rich in essential vitamins, minerals, antioxidants, and phytonutrients that support optimal health and immune function.

- Unlike processed foods, which may undergo nutrient degradation during manufacturing and storage, fresh foods retain their nutritional integrity, offering a wealth of bioavailable nutrients to nourish the body.

3. Enhanced Digestibility:

- Whole foods are often easier for the body to digest and assimilate compared to highly processed or refined foods laden with additives and preservatives.

- The fiber content in whole fruits, vegetables, and grains supports digestive health by promoting regularity, optimizing nutrient absorption, and fostering a healthy gut microbiome.

4. Reduced Chemical Exposure:

- Fresh and whole foods are less likely to contain synthetic additives, artificial flavors, and chemical preservatives commonly found in processed foods.

- By choosing organic and locally sourced options whenever possible, individuals minimize their exposure to pesticides, herbicides, and other potentially harmful chemicals present in conventionally grown produce.

5. Diverse Nutritional Profile:

- Incorporating a variety of fresh fruits, vegetables, whole grains, legumes, nuts, seeds, and lean proteins ensures a diverse nutritional profile, providing the body with a spectrum of essential nutrients and micronutrients.

- Phytochemicals and bioactive compounds found abundantly in fresh produce offer protective benefits against inflammation, oxidative stress, and chronic disease.

6. Supporting Immune Function:

- Fresh and whole foods supply the body with the building blocks it needs to maintain a robust immune system and mount an effective defense against pathogens and environmental stressors.

- Nutrient-dense foods, such as leafy greens, berries, citrus fruits, and omega-3 fatty acids from oily fish, bolster immune function and help modulate inflammatory responses.

7. Promoting Long-Term Health and Vitality:

- Adopting a diet rich in fresh and whole foods contributes to long-term health and vitality, reducing the risk of chronic diseases such as cardiovascular disease, diabetes, obesity, and certain cancers.

- By nourishing the body with wholesome, nutrient-rich foods, individuals lay the foundation for sustained energy, mental clarity, and overall vitality throughout the lifespan.

In essence, embracing fresh and whole foods empowers individuals with histamine intolerance to nourish their bodies, support their immune systems, and thrive in the face of dietary challenges. By prioritizing nutrient-dense options and cultivating a mindful approach to food selection and preparation, individuals harness the healing power of nature's bounty and reclaim control over their health and well-being.

- Balancing Macronutrients for Histamine Sensitivity

For individuals navigating histamine sensitivity, achieving a well-rounded diet that balances macronutrients is essential for managing symptoms, supporting overall health, and promoting vitality. Here's a closer look at how to optimize macronutrient intake in the context of histamine sensitivity:

1. Proteins:

- **Quality Sources:** Prioritize lean, high-quality protein sources such as poultry, fish, eggs, legumes, tofu, and tempeh. Opt for fresh, unprocessed options whenever possible to minimize histamine content.

- **Moderation:** While protein is essential for muscle repair, immune function, and hormone regulation, excessive intake can strain the body's detoxification pathways and potentially exacerbate histamine sensitivity. Aim for a balanced intake of protein throughout the day rather than relying heavily on protein-rich foods in one meal.

2. Carbohydrates:

- **Complex Carbs:** Choose complex carbohydrates from whole grains, fruits, vegetables, and legumes to provide sustained energy and support digestive health. Whole grains like quinoa, brown rice, oats, and barley offer fiber, vitamins, and minerals while minimizing blood sugar spikes.

- **Limit Refined Sugars:** Minimize consumption of refined sugars and processed carbohydrates, which can contribute to inflammation and disrupt blood sugar balance. When choosing sweeteners, go for natural options like dates, honey, or maple syrup.

3. Fats:

- **Healthy Fats:** Incorporate sources of healthy fats such as avocados, nuts, seeds, olive oil, and fatty fish like salmon and mackerel. These fats provide essential omega-3 and omega-6 fatty acids, which support brain function, hormone production, and cardiovascular health.

- **Omega-3 Supplementation:** Consider omega-3 supplementation if dietary intake is insufficient. Omega-3 fatty acids have anti-inflammatory properties and may help alleviate symptoms of histamine intolerance.

4. Hydration:

- **Water Intake:** Stay adequately hydrated by drinking plenty of water throughout the day. Proper hydration supports detoxification, aids digestion, and helps maintain electrolyte balance.

- **Herbal Teas:** Enjoy herbal teas like chamomile, peppermint, and ginger, which are hydrating and may have soothing effects on the digestive system. Avoid teas containing high-histamine herbs like nettle or hibiscus if they trigger symptoms.

5. Meal Timing and Frequency:

- **Regular Meals:** Aim for regular, balanced meals spaced evenly throughout the day to stabilize blood sugar levels and prevent energy crashes.

- **Snack Options:** Incorporate healthy snacks like fresh fruit, raw vegetables with hummus, or a handful of nuts to maintain energy levels between meals. Choose low-histamine options to minimize the risk of triggering symptoms.

6. Individualized Approach:

- **Listen to Your Body:** Pay attention to how different macronutrient ratios and food combinations affect your symptoms. Keep a food diary to track your dietary intake and any associated reactions, helping identify patterns and potential triggers.

- **Work with a Professional:** Consider consulting a registered dietitian or healthcare provider specializing in histamine intolerance for personalized dietary guidance. They can help tailor a nutrition plan that meets your individual needs and supports your health goals.

7. Mindful Eating:

- **Savor Each Bite:** Practice mindful eating by slowing down, savoring each bite, and paying attention to hunger and fullness cues. Chew food thoroughly to aid digestion and optimize nutrient absorption.

- **Reduce Stress:** Minimize stress during mealtime to support proper digestion and assimilation of nutrients. Engage in relaxation techniques like deep breathing, meditation, or gentle stretching before and after meals.

Balancing Macronutrient Ratios:

1. **Individualized Approach:** Tailor macronutrient ratios to suit your unique dietary needs, metabolic profile, and activity levels. Experiment with different proportions of proteins, fats, and carbohydrates to find the optimal balance that supports your health goals and histamine sensitivity.
2. **Monitor Response:** Pay attention to how your body responds to different macronutrient compositions. Adjust your diet accordingly based on changes in energy levels, digestive comfort, and overall well-being.
3. **Consultation with a Professional:** Seek guidance from a registered dietitian or healthcare provider specializing in histamine intolerance to develop a personalized nutrition plan. They can offer expert advice, monitor your progress, and make recommendations based on your specific dietary requirements and health status.

Chapter 3

Building Your Anti-Histamine Diet Plan

- **Sample Meal Plans and Recipes**

Managing histamine sensitivity requires thoughtful planning and mindful selection of foods to minimize symptom flare-ups while ensuring optimal nutrition. Sample meal plans tailored to histamine sensitivity can help individuals navigate their dietary needs effectively. Here's a glimpse into a day's worth of nourishing meals:

Sample Meal Plan:

Breakfast:

- **Quinoa Breakfast Bowl:**

  - Cooked quinoa as the base.

  - Topped with sliced avocado, diced cucumber, and cherry tomatoes.

  - Garnished with a squeeze of lemon juice and olive oil.Garnished with chopped fresh herbs like parsley or basil.

Mid-Morning Snack:

- **Green Smoothie:**

    - Blend together fresh spinach, cucumber, pineapple, and coconut water.

    - Optionally add a scoop of pea protein powder or a handful of hemp seeds for added protein.

Lunch:

- **Grilled Salmon Salad:**

    - Grilled salmon fillet served over a bed of mixed greens (e.g., arugula, spinach).

    - Tossed with sliced strawberries, toasted walnuts, and crumbled goat cheese (optional).

    - Drizzled with a balsamic vinaigrette made with olive oil, balsamic vinegar, Dijon mustard, and honey (or maple syrup for sweetness).

Afternoon Snack:

- **Celery Sticks with Almond Butter:**

    - Fresh celery sticks paired with creamy almond butter for a satisfying and nutrient-rich snack.

Dinner:

- **Turkey and Vegetable Stir-Fry:**

    - Sautéed ground turkey with garlic, ginger, and chopped vegetables (bell peppers, broccoli, snap peas) in a sesame oil stir-fry sauce (tamari, rice vinegar, honey).

    - Served over a bed of cauliflower rice or quinoa for a wholesome and filling meal.

Evening Snack:

- **Mixed Berries with Coconut Yogurt:**

    - Assorted fresh berries (strawberries, blueberries, raspberries) served with dairy-free coconut yogurt for a refreshing and antioxidant-rich dessert.

Key Considerations:

- **Focus on Freshness:** Incorporate fresh, whole foods whenever possible to minimize histamine exposure and maximize nutrient content.

- **Colorful Plate:** Aim for a variety of colorful fruits and vegetables to ensure a diverse range of vitamins, minerals, and phytonutrients.

- **Hydration:** Stay hydrated throughout the day by drinking plenty of water, herbal teas, and infused water with slices of citrus or cucumber.

- **Mindful Portions:** Pay attention to portion sizes and listen to your body's hunger and fullness cues to avoid overeating and promote digestive comfort.

- **Individual Adaptations:** Customize meal plans based on personal preferences, dietary restrictions, and tolerance levels to ensure a sustainable and enjoyable eating experience.

- Grocery Shopping Guide for Low-Histamine Foods

For individuals managing histamine intolerance, navigating the grocery store can be a daunting task. However, armed with knowledge and a strategic approach, you can confidently fill your cart with low-histamine foods to support your dietary needs. Here's a comprehensive grocery shopping guide to help you make informed choices:

1. Fresh Produce Section:

- **Vegetables:** Opt for fresh, non-canned vegetables such as spinach, kale, cucumber, carrots, broccoli, cauliflower, bell peppers, and zucchini.

- **Fruits:** Choose low-histamine fruits like apples, pears, berries (strawberries, blueberries, raspberries), cherries, grapes, melons, and citrus fruits (lemons, limes, oranges).

2. Meat and Poultry:

- **Fresh Meat:** Select fresh cuts of meat and poultry, including chicken, turkey, beef, pork, and lamb. Avoid processed and cured meats, as they may contain higher levels of histamine.

- **Fish:** Opt for fresh fish varieties such as salmon, cod, haddock, trout, and sole. Avoid smoked, canned, and aged fish, which tend to be higher in histamine.

3. Dairy and Alternatives:

- **Fresh Dairy:** Choose fresh dairy products such as milk, yogurt, and cheese made from pasteurized milk. Opt for varieties with shorter fermentation times and lower histamine levels.

- **Non-Dairy Alternatives:** Explore non-dairy options like almond milk, coconut milk, rice milk, and oat milk. Look for unsweetened and unflavored varieties to minimize histamine exposure.

4. Grains and Legumes:

- **Whole Grains:** Stock up on whole grains like rice (white, brown, basmati), quinoa, millet, oats, and buckwheat. These grains are naturally low in histamine and rich in fiber and nutrients.

- **Legumes:** Choose legumes such as lentils, chickpeas, black beans, and mung beans for protein and fiber.

Soak and cook them thoroughly to reduce histamine content.

5. Nuts and Seeds:

- **Fresh Nuts:** Select fresh nuts like almonds, walnuts, pecans, and cashews. Avoid nuts that have been roasted, salted, or processed, as they may contain additives and higher histamine levels.

- **Seeds:** Add seeds such as chia seeds, flaxseeds, pumpkin seeds, and sunflower seeds to your shopping list for added nutrition and texture.

6. Condiments and Cooking Ingredients:

- **Oils:** Choose cold-pressed oils like olive oil, coconut oil, and avocado oil for cooking and dressing. Avoid processed oils and margarine, which may contain additives and preservatives.

- **Herbs and Spices:** Use fresh herbs like parsley, basil, cilantro, and chives to season dishes. Limit the use of dried herbs and spices, as they may contain higher levels of histamine.

- **Vinegar:** Opt for apple cider vinegar or white vinegar as low-histamine alternatives to other types of vinegar like balsamic and red wine vinegar.

7. Frozen Foods:

- **Frozen Vegetables and Fruits:** Keep your freezer stocked with frozen vegetables and fruits for convenience and freshness. Choose plain frozen options without added sauces or seasonings.

- **Frozen Fish and Seafood:** Consider purchasing frozen fish and seafood varieties to have on hand for quick and easy meals. Look for options labeled as fresh-frozen with no added preservatives.

8. Beverages:

- **Water:** Stay hydrated with filtered water as your primary beverage choice. Avoid carbonated drinks, energy drinks, and alcoholic beverages, which may contain higher levels of histamine.

- **Herbal Teas:** Enjoy a variety of caffeine-free herbal teas such as chamomile, peppermint, ginger, and rooibos for hydration and relaxation.

9. Baked Goods and Snacks:

- **Gluten-Free Options:** Explore gluten-free baked goods and snacks made with low-histamine ingredients like rice flour, tapioca flour, and almond flour.

- **Homemade Treats:** Consider baking your own treats using low-histamine ingredients and natural sweeteners like honey, maple syrup, or coconut sugar to control the quality of ingredients.

10. Specialty Foods and Ethnic Aisles:

- **International Flavors:** Explore the ethnic aisles for ingredients used in cuisines with naturally low-histamine profiles, such as Asian, Mediterranean, and Middle Eastern cuisines.

- **Coconut-Based Products:** Look for coconut-based products like coconut milk, coconut cream, and coconut flour as alternatives to dairy and wheat-based ingredients.

11. Fresh Herbs and Spices:

- **Grow Your Own:** Consider growing your own fresh herbs at home to ensure a steady supply of flavorful additions to your meals. Herbs like basil, mint, and cilantro thrive in small indoor herb gardens.

- **Minimal Processing:** Opt for fresh herbs and spices over pre-packaged options, as they are less likely to contain additives and preservatives that can trigger histamine reactions.

12. Meal Planning and List-Making:

- **Plan Ahead:** Create a weekly meal plan and shopping list based on low-histamine recipes and ingredients. This helps streamline your shopping experience and ensures you have everything you need for nutritious meals throughout the week.

- **Stick to Your List:** Stay focused on purchasing items from your list to avoid impulse buys and minimize exposure to high-histamine foods that may tempt you while browsing the aisles.

13. Online Resources and Delivery Services:

- **Online Shopping:** Take advantage of online grocery shopping and delivery services that offer a wide selection of low-histamine products. This convenient option allows you to shop from the comfort of your home and access specialty items that may not be available at local stores.

- **Subscription Boxes:** Explore subscription box services specializing in health-conscious and allergy-friendly foods, which often feature curated selections of low-histamine products tailored to specific dietary needs.

14. Read Labels and Ingredients:

- **Know Your Ingredients:** Familiarize yourself with common ingredients and additives that may trigger histamine reactions, such as artificial colors, flavors, and preservatives.

- **Check Expiry Dates:** Pay attention to expiry dates and freshness indicators when selecting perishable items like meat, dairy, and produce to ensure optimal quality and minimize histamine formation.

- ## Strategies for Dining Out and Social Events

Managing histamine sensitivity goes beyond the constraints of home cooking, creating distinct issues when dining out or attending social events. However, with smart preparation and great communication, you may enjoy eating events while avoiding histamine exposure. Here are some practical techniques to negotiate eating out and social events:

1. Research Restaurants in Advance:
- *Check Menus Online*: Review restaurant menus online to locate low-histamine alternatives and plan your meal selections ahead of time.
- *Choose Restaurants Wisely*: Opt for restaurants recognised for their fresh, made-to-order cuisine and flexibility in addressing dietary requirements.

2. Communicate with Restaurant Staff:

- *Inform Servers*: Communicate your dietary demands and histamine sensitivity to your server or the restaurant staff. Request alterations to meals or replacements to fit your preferences.
- *Ask Questions*: Don't hesitate to inquire about ingredients, cooking techniques, and possible sources of histamine in foods. Seek clarification to ensure your food matches with your dietary limitations.

3. Focus on Simple, Fresh Options:

- ***Stick to Basics***: Choose basic, unprocessed foods with fresh ingredients like salads, grilled meats or seafood, steamed veggies, and plain rice or potatoes.
- ***Avoid Sauces and Marinades***: Request sauces, dressings, and marinades on the side or ask about low-histamine alternatives. Opt for olive oil and vinegar or lemon juice as lighter choices.

4. Be Mindful of Preparation Methods:

- ***Opt for Grilled or Steamed***: Select foods that are grilled, steamed, or sautéed with minimum spice to limit the chance of histamine buildup during cooking.
- ***Avoid Deep-Fried and Aged Foods***: Steer away of deep-fried goods and aged meats, cheeses, and fermented foods, which may have greater amounts of histamine.

5. BYO selections: Bring Your Own Ingredients:

- Consider bringing low-histamine snacks or condiments to social gatherings or restaurants to enhance your meal selections and ensure you have adequate alternatives available.
- ***Pack Emergency Snacks***: Carry portable, non-perishable snacks like almonds, seeds, fruit, or rice cakes to have on hand in case acceptable meal alternatives are limited.

6. Practice Portion Control and Moderation:

- *Listen to Your Body*: Pay attention to portion sizes and how your body reacts to various meals. Avoid overindulging in high-histamine goods to limit the chance of unpleasant responses.
- *Prioritize Quality over Quantity*: Focus on appreciating smaller servings of high-quality, nutrient-dense meals to please your taste while supporting your nutritional objectives.

7. Plan Ahead for Social Events:

- *Communicate with Hosts*: Inform hosts or event organizers about your histamine sensitivity and dietary demands in advance. Offer to provide a meal or propose low-histamine food ideas to fit your needs.
- *Scope Out the Menu*: If attending a catered event or gathering at a restaurant, ask about menu selections and suggest alterations or alternatives if required.

8. Mindful Eating Practices:
- *Slow Down and Enjoy:* Practice mindful eating by enjoying each mouthful, chewing gently, and paying attention to tastes, textures, and sensations.

- *Stay Present:* Focus on the social side of eating out and connecting with companions, rather than focusing on the food. Enjoy the company and discussion while fueling your body with proper options.

By applying these tactics and speaking for your dietary requirements, you may negotiate eating out and social occasions with confidence and have significant culinary experiences while managing histamine sensitivity. Remember to promote open communication, flexibility, and self-care to make meal events joyful and inclusive for everyone involved.

Chapter 4

Lifestyle Factors and Histamine Intolerance

- Stress Management Techniques

Living with histamine sensitivity may be tough since stress typically exacerbates symptoms and undermines general well-being. Implementing proactive stress management practices may help people deal with the demands of everyday life while avoiding histamine-related symptoms. Here are many ways to consider:

1. Mindfulness Meditation:

- **Practice Daily Meditation**: Set aside devoted time each day for mindfulness meditation to quiet the mind, lower stress levels, and build a feeling of inner serenity.
- **Focus on the Present Moment**: Engage in mindfulness techniques that increase present-moment awareness, such as deep breathing, body scanning, and guided imagery.

2. Deep Breathing Exercises:

- Diaphragmatic Breathing: Practice deep breathing methods to trigger the body's relaxation response and counteract the physiological consequences of stress. Focus on calm, rhythmic breaths that expand the diaphragm and encourage relaxation.

- Incorporate Breathing pauses: Take small pauses throughout the day to participate in deep breathing exercises, especially during periods of heightened stress or tension.

3. Physical Activity and Exercise:

- Choose Gentle Activities: Engage in low-impact activities such as yoga, tai chi, strolling, or swimming to induce relaxation, release stress, and enhance general well-being.

- Prioritize Consistency: Establish a regular exercise regimen that matches your schedule and preferences, aiming for at least 30 minutes of moderate activity most days of the week.

4. Mind-Body Practices:
- Yoga and Pilates: Participate in yoga or Pilates sessions that emphasize gentle movements, stretching,

and mindfulness methods to develop body awareness and promote stress alleviation.

- Progressive Muscle Relaxation: Practice progressive muscle relaxation techniques to gradually tension and release muscle groups throughout the body, producing physical and mental calm.

5. Healthy Lifestyle Habits:

- Prioritize Sleep: Maintain a regular sleep schedule and establish a pleasant sleep environment favorable to relaxation and renewal. Aim for 7-9 hours of decent sleep each night.

- Nutrition and Hydration: Fuel your body with good, low-histamine meals and remain hydrated throughout the day to promote optimum physical and mental performance.

6. Cultivate Supportive Relationships:

- Reach Out for Support: Connect with friends, family members, or support groups that understand and sympathize with your histamine sensitivity journey. Share your experiences and get emotional assistance when required.

- Engage in Meaningful Activities: Participate in social activities, hobbies, and interests that offer pleasure, satisfaction, and a feeling of belonging.

6. *Time Management and Boundaries:*
- Set Realistic Goals: Prioritize chores and responsibilities, creating manageable objectives while keeping realistic expectations for yourself.

- Establish Boundaries: Learn to say no to excessive commitments and duties that lead to stress and overload. Honor your limitations and fight for your needs.

- Sleep and Exercise for Histamine Sensitivity

Balanced sleep patterns and regular physical exercise play crucial roles in controlling histamine sensitivity and supporting general well-being. Implementing good sleep patterns and participating in proper exercise routines may help reduce symptoms, increase immune function, and improve quality of life. Here are techniques to maximize sleep and exercise for those with histamine sensitivity:

Sleep Management:

Establish a Consistent Sleep Schedule:

- Aim to maintain a normal sleep-wake cycle by going to bed and getting up at the same time each day, especially on weekends.
- Consistency helps regulate circadian rhythms and supports restorative sleep patterns.

Create a Restful Sleep Environment:

- Design your bedroom for maximum sleep by keeping it cool, dark, and quiet.
- Consider utilizing blackout curtains, white noise generators, or earplugs to limit disturbances and create a suitable sleep environment.

Limit Exposure to Stimulants and Electronic Devices:

- Avoid coffee, nicotine, and stimulating activities close to bedtime, since these may interfere with sleep onset and quality.
- Reduce screen time and exposure to blue light from electronic devices at least an hour before sleep to encourage natural melatonin synthesis.

Practice Relaxation Techniques:

- Wind down before bed with peaceful activities such as reading, moderate stretching, meditation, or deep breathing exercises.
- Incorporate relaxation methods into your nightly routine to communicate to your body that it's time to unwind and prepare for sleep.

Address Underlying Sleep Disorders:

- If you have chronic sleep disruptions or insomnia, speak with a healthcare practitioner to assess and manage underlying sleep problems, such as sleep apnea, restless legs syndrome, or insomnia.

Exercise Guidelines:

Choose Low-Impact Activities:

- Opt for low-impact workouts like walking, cycling, swimming, or moderate yoga to decrease stress on joints and muscles while increasing cardiovascular health and flexibility.
- Select activities that you love and can continue over time without increasing histamine-related symptoms.

Gradually Increase Intensity and Duration:

- Start with shorter training sessions and progressively increase intensity and length as your fitness level increases.
- Listen to your body's cues and adapt your exercise intensity or length to prevent overexertion and limit the danger of histamine responses.

Incorporate Strength Training and Flexibility Exercises:

- Include strength training exercises utilizing body weight, resistance bands, or small weights to increase muscular strength and promote joint stability.
- Incorporate flexibility exercises and stretching regimens to enhance range of motion, decrease muscular tension, and avoid injuries.

Be Mindful of Environmental Triggers:

- Choose workout areas with acceptable air quality and limited exposure to allergens, pollution, and irritants that may induce histamine sensitivity.
- Consider indoor choices during high pollen or pollution seasons to limit possible allergy exposure during outside activities.

Listen to Your Body:

- Pay attention to how your body reacts to exercise and alter your regimen appropriately.
- Honor your energy levels and rest when required, providing appropriate time for recuperation and regeneration between sessions.

- Environmental Triggers to Avoid

For individuals with histamine sensitivity, minimizing exposure to environmental triggers is essential for managing symptoms and maintaining optimal health. Being mindful of potential triggers in the environment can help mitigate histamine-related reactions and promote overall well-being. Here are common environmental triggers to avoid:

1. Allergens:

- **Pollen and Mold:** Limit exposure to outdoor allergens such as pollen and mold spores, especially during high pollen seasons or in damp, mold-prone environments.

- **Dust Mites:** Take steps to reduce dust mites in indoor spaces by using allergen-proof mattress and pillow covers, vacuuming regularly, and maintaining low humidity levels.

2. Airborne Irritants:

- **Smoke and Pollution:** Avoid exposure to tobacco smoke, vehicle emissions, and industrial pollutants, which can exacerbate respiratory symptoms and trigger histamine reactions.

- **Strong Odors:** Steer clear of strong chemical odors, perfumes, air fresheners, and household cleaning products that may contain volatile organic compounds (VOCs) known to induce histamine release.

3. Food Allergens and Sensitivities:

- **High-Histamine Foods:** Identify and avoid foods that are high in histamine content or that trigger histamine release in sensitive individuals. Common culprits include aged cheeses, fermented foods, processed meats, and alcoholic beverages.

- **Food Additives:** Be cautious of food additives such as artificial preservatives, flavor enhancers (e.g., monosodium glutamate), and artificial colors, which can exacerbate histamine sensitivity in some individuals.

4. Temperature and Humidity Extremes:

- **Extreme Temperatures:** Minimize exposure to extreme heat or cold, as temperature fluctuations can trigger histamine-related symptoms in susceptible individuals.

- **High Humidity:** Be mindful of indoor humidity levels, as excessive moisture can promote mold growth and allergen accumulation. Use dehumidifiers and proper ventilation to maintain optimal indoor air quality.

5. Stress and Emotional Triggers:

- **Psychological Stress:** Manage stress through relaxation techniques, mindfulness practices, and stress-reducing activities to prevent the release of stress hormones that can exacerbate histamine sensitivity.

- **Emotional Triggers:** Identify and address emotional triggers such as anxiety, anger, or sadness that may contribute to histamine-related symptoms. Seek support from mental health professionals or support groups as needed.

6. Insect Stings and Bites:

- **Avoidance Measures:** Take precautions to avoid insect stings and bites by wearing protective clothing, using insect repellents, and avoiding areas with high insect activity, especially during peak seasons.

- **Prompt Treatment:** If stung or bitten, promptly remove the stinger (if applicable) and apply appropriate first aid measures to reduce inflammation and minimize histamine release.

7. Medication and Chemical Sensitivities:

- **Medication Allergies:** Be aware of potential medication allergies and adverse reactions, including those related to over-the-counter medications, antibiotics, and nonsteroidal anti-inflammatory drugs (NSAIDs).

- **Chemical Sensitivities:** Minimize exposure to chemicals, solvents, and environmental toxins found in personal care products, cosmetics, and household cleaners. Opt for fragrance-free, hypoallergenic alternatives whenever possible.

By proactively identifying and avoiding environmental triggers, individuals with histamine sensitivity can reduce the frequency and severity of symptoms, improve quality of life, and better manage their condition.

Chapter 5

Supplements and Natural Remedies

- **Vitamins and Minerals to Support Histamine Metabolism**

Histamine metabolism is a complex process involving various enzymes and cofactors that help regulate histamine levels in the body. Certain vitamins and minerals play critical roles in supporting histamine metabolism and promoting optimal functioning of histamine-related pathways. Here are key nutrients that can support histamine metabolism:

1. Vitamin C:

- **Role:** Vitamin C acts as a natural antihistamine and antioxidant, helping to stabilize mast cells and reduce histamine release.

- **Food Sources:** Citrus fruits (oranges, lemons, limes), strawberries, kiwi, bell peppers, broccoli, and leafy greens.

2. Vitamin B6 (Pyridoxine):

- **Role:** Vitamin B6 is involved in the conversion of histidine (an amino acid) to histamine and helps regulate histamine levels in the body.

- **Food Sources:** Chicken, turkey, fish, potatoes, bananas, chickpeas, sunflower seeds, and fortified cereals.

3. Vitamin B12 (Cobalamin):

- **Role:** Vitamin B12 supports methylation processes involved in histamine metabolism and may help modulate histamine levels.

- **Food Sources:** Animal products such as meat, fish, eggs, and dairy, as well as fortified plant-based foods like nutritional yeast and some cereals.

4. Magnesium:

- **Role:** Magnesium supports the activity of DAO (diamine oxidase), an enzyme responsible for breaking down histamine in the gut.

- **Food Sources:** Spinach, kale, Swiss chard, almonds, cashews, avocado, bananas, and legumes (beans, lentils).

5. Zinc:

- **Role:** Zinc is involved in the regulation of histamine release from mast cells and supports the functioning of histamine receptors.

- **Food Sources:** Oysters, red meat, poultry, seafood, pumpkin seeds, sesame seeds, chickpeas, and lentils.

6. Quercetin:

- **Role:** Quercetin is a flavonoid with anti-inflammatory properties that may help stabilize mast cells and inhibit histamine release.

- **Food Sources:** Apples, onions, citrus fruits, berries, grapes, capers, parsley, kale, and broccoli.

7. Omega-3 Fatty Acids:

- **Role:** Omega-3 fatty acids help modulate inflammatory responses and may reduce the production of pro-inflammatory histamine.

- **Food Sources:** Fatty fish (salmon, mackerel, sardines), flaxseeds, chia seeds, walnuts, hemp seeds, and algae-based supplements.

8. Probiotics:

- **Role:** Probiotics promote gut health and may help maintain the balance of gut bacteria involved in histamine metabolism and immune regulation.

- **Food Sources:** Fermented foods such as yogurt, kefir, sauerkraut, kimchi, miso, and kombucha.

9. Copper:

- **Role:** Copper is a cofactor for DAO enzyme activity, which is essential for breaking down histamine in the digestive tract.

- **Food Sources:** Organ meats (liver, kidneys), shellfish (oysters, crab), nuts (cashews, almonds), seeds (sesame, sunflower), and cocoa.

10. Selenium:

- **Role:** Selenium supports antioxidant defenses and may help regulate immune responses related to histamine release.

- **Food Sources:** Brazil nuts, seafood (oysters, tuna, shrimp), sunflower seeds, eggs, and mushrooms.

- Herbal Remedies for Allergy Relief

Herbal remedies have been used for centuries to alleviate allergy symptoms and promote respiratory health. While research on their effectiveness varies, many herbs are believed to possess anti-inflammatory, antihistamine, and immune-modulating properties that may provide relief from allergy symptoms. Here are some herbal remedies commonly used for allergy relief:

1. Nettle (Urtica dioica):

- **Benefits:** Nettle is rich in bioactive compounds that may help reduce allergic inflammation and histamine release.

- **Forms:** Nettle leaf can be consumed as tea, tincture, or capsules. It can also be used fresh or dried in cooking.

2. Butterbur (Petasites hybridus):

- **Benefits:** Butterbur extract may help alleviate allergic rhinitis symptoms by reducing inflammation and blocking histamine receptors.

- **Forms:** Butterbur supplements are available in capsules or tablets. Ensure the product is labeled "PA-free" to avoid potential liver toxicity.

3. Quercetin:

- **Benefits:** Quercetin is a flavonoid with antioxidant and anti-inflammatory properties that may help stabilize mast cells and reduce histamine release.

- **Sources:** Found naturally in foods like onions, apples, citrus fruits, berries, and leafy greens. Also available in supplement form.

4. Turmeric (Curcuma longa):

- **Benefits:** Turmeric contains curcumin, a compound known for its anti-inflammatory and immune-modulating effects, which may help alleviate allergy symptoms.

- **Forms:** Turmeric can be consumed as a spice in cooking, taken as a supplement, or consumed as turmeric tea.

5. Ginger (Zingiber officinale):

- **Benefits:** Ginger has anti-inflammatory and antioxidant properties that may help alleviate allergy symptoms, including nasal congestion and respiratory discomfort.

- **Forms:** Fresh ginger can be grated and steeped to make tea.

6. Echinacea (Echinacea purpurea):

- **Benefits:** Echinacea is believed to support immune function and reduce the severity and duration of upper respiratory tract infections, including those related to allergies.

- **Forms:** Echinacea supplements are available in capsules, tablets, and tinctures.

7. Licorice Root (Glycyrrhiza glabra):

- **Benefits:** Licorice root has anti-inflammatory and antiviral properties that may help soothe irritated mucous membranes and alleviate allergy symptoms.

- **Forms:** Licorice root tea, capsules, or tinctures are commonly used for allergy relief.

8. Peppermint (Mentha piperita):

- **Benefits:** Peppermint contains menthol, which can help relieve nasal congestion and soothe irritated airways associated with allergies.

- **Forms:** Peppermint tea, essential oil (for aromatherapy or steam inhalation), or capsules.

9. Ginkgo Biloba:

- **Benefits:** Ginkgo biloba extract may have anti-inflammatory and antioxidant properties that help reduce allergy symptoms and improve circulation.

- **Forms:** Ginkgo biloba supplements are available in capsule or tablet form.

10. Chamomile (Matricaria chamomilla):

- **Benefits:** Chamomile has anti-inflammatory and antihistamine properties that may help alleviate allergy symptoms and promote relaxation.

- **Forms:** Chamomile tea, capsules, or essential oil for aromatherapy.

While herbal remedies can offer relief for some individuals, it's important to consult with a healthcare professional before starting any herbal treatment, especially if you have underlying health conditions or are taking medications. Additionally, be aware of potential allergies or interactions with other medications when using herbal supplements.

■ Probiotics and Gut Health

Understanding the Connection Between Probiotics and Gut Health with Probiotics

The microbiome of the gut, which is made up of billions of bacteria that live in the gastrointestinal system, is an extremely important component in the process of preserving people's general health and well-being. There is evidence that probiotics, which are helpful bacteria that may be found in some foods and supplements, can help maintain healthy gut flora and contribute to a variety of physiological processes. An investigation of the relationship between probiotics and the health of the gut is presented here:

- Probiotics help maintain a healthy balance of beneficial bacteria in the gut, which is needed for normal digestion, nutrient absorption, and immunological function. Another benefit of probiotics is that they assist preserve microbial equilibrium.
- -! As a result of their competition with hazardous pathogens for resources and space, they can suppress the development of harmful bacteria and avoid dysbiosis, which is classified as an imbalance of microorganisms.

2. Enhancing Digestive Function:

- Probiotics create enzymes that help in the breakdown of carbs, proteins, and lipids, promoting effective digestion and nutrient absorption. –
- In addition to this, they assist in the regulation of bowel motions and the alleviation of symptoms associated with digestive diseases such as irritable bowel syndrome (IBS) and constipation.

3. Supporting Immune Function:

- A large percentage of the body's immune system is situated in the gut-associated lymphoid tissue (GALT), where probiotics interact with immune cells and modify immunological responses.
- Probiotics help strengthen the intestinal barrier, reducing the passage of toxic chemicals and pathogens into the circulation.

4. Reducing Inflammation:

- Certain strains of probiotics have anti-inflammatory capabilities and may help alleviate chronic inflammation in the stomach and other regions of the body.
- It has been suggested that probiotics may improve symptoms of inflammatory bowel disorders (IBD) and other inflammatory ailments. This is accomplished via the regulation of inflammatory cytokines and the promotion of immunological tolerance.

5. *Improving Mental Health:*
- The gut-brain axis, a bidirectional communication network between the stomach and the brain, plays a critical role in mental health and emotional well-being.
- Probiotics increase neurotransmitter synthesis, control stress hormones, and modify brain pathways, possibly improving mood disorders such as sadness and anxiety.

6. *Managing Allergic Reactions:*
- Probiotics help control immune responses and minimize the risk of allergic reactions by improving immunological tolerance and modifying inflammatory pathways.
- They may be especially effective in avoiding or treating symptoms of allergic rhinitis, eczema, and food allergies.

7. *Enhancing Nutrient Absorption:*
- Probiotics boost the bioavailability of certain nutrients, including vitamins, minerals, and phytonutrients, by promoting their absorption and use in the gut.
- They also assist in metabolizing food components and transforming them into bioactive forms that are more easily absorbed by the body.

8. Supporting Metabolic Health:

- Emerging evidence shows that probiotics may have a role in metabolic health by affecting glucose metabolism, lipid profile, and body weight management.
- Certain probiotic strains have been related to improvements in insulin sensitivity, cholesterol levels, and indicators of metabolic syndrome.

Incorporating probiotic-rich foods such as yogurt, kefir, sauerkraut, kimchi, and kombucha into your diet will help build a healthy gut microbiota. Additionally, probiotic pills containing particular strains may be effective for treating certain health conditions or improving general gut health. However, it's vital to purchase high-quality probiotic products with evidence-based strains and speak with a healthcare practitioner for specific recommendations targeted to your unique requirements and health objectives. By feeding your gut microbiota with probiotics and adopting a balanced diet rich in fiber and minerals, you may improve digestive function, promote immunological resilience, and increase overall health and vitality.

Chapter 6

Tracking Progress and Managing Symptoms

Keeping a Food and Symptom Journal

Keeping a food and symptom journal is a valuable tool for identifying potential triggers, understanding patterns, and managing various health conditions, including allergies, intolerances, digestive disorders, and autoimmune diseases. Here's a guide on how to maintain a food and symptom journal effectively:

1. Choose a Format:

- Select a journal format that suits your preferences and lifestyle. Options include traditional notebooks, digital apps, or online templates specifically designed for tracking food intake and symptoms.

2. Record Food Intake:

- Write down everything you eat and drink throughout the day, including portion sizes, ingredients, and cooking methods. Be as detailed as possible to accurately capture your dietary habits.

3. Document Symptoms:

- Record any symptoms or reactions you experience, such as bloating, abdominal pain, fatigue, headaches, skin rashes, or respiratory issues. Note the severity, duration, and timing of each symptom.

4. Note Timing and Context:

- Document the time of day when you consume meals and snacks, as well as any relevant contextual factors such as stress levels, physical activity, medication use, and environmental exposures.

5. Be Consistent:

- Make journaling a daily habit to ensure consistency and accuracy in tracking your food intake and symptoms. Set aside dedicated time each day to update your journal and reflect on your observations.

6. Use Descriptive Language:

- Use descriptive language to describe your symptoms and how they impact your daily life. Include details about the intensity, location, and specific characteristics of each symptom.

7. Identify Patterns:

- Review your journal entries regularly to identify potential patterns or correlations between your food choices and symptoms. Look for trends in symptom onset, duration, and severity in relation to specific foods or beverages.

8. Experiment with Elimination:

- Consider conducting structured elimination diets or removing suspected trigger foods from your diet based on your journal findings. Monitor changes in symptoms and assess the effectiveness of dietary modifications over time.

9. Seek Professional Guidance:

- Consult with a healthcare professional, registered dietitian, or allergist for guidance and support in interpreting your journal data, identifying trigger foods, and developing personalized dietary strategies.

10. Be Patient and Persistent:

- Recognize that identifying food triggers and managing symptoms may require time, patience, and perseverance. Be open to experimentation and willing to adapt your approach based on ongoing observations and feedback.

11. Monitor Progress:

- Track your progress over time and celebrate small victories along the way. Notice improvements in symptoms, energy levels, and overall well-being as you make informed dietary changes and lifestyle adjustments.

12. Stay Mindful and Reflective:

- Use your food and symptom journal as a tool for self-awareness and mindfulness. Pay attention to how different foods and lifestyle factors affect your body and emotions, and make informed choices accordingly.

Maintaining a food and symptom journal empowers you to take an active role in managing your health and making informed decisions about your diet and lifestyle. By fostering greater awareness of your body's responses to various foods and environmental factors, you can optimize your nutrition, minimize discomfort, and enhance your overall quality of life.

Recognizing Flare-Ups and Managing Reactions

1. ***Know Your Triggers:*** Identify typical triggers that increase your symptoms, such as particular meals, environmental allergies, stresses, hormone fluctuations, or lifestyle variables.

Keep a careful note of your triggers and analyze trends in symptom flare-ups to better understand your body's responses.

2. ***Recognize Early Warning Signs***: Pay attention to minor changes in your body and emotions that may signify an upcoming flare-up or response.

Common early warning indicators include weariness, mood changes, stomach pain, skin irritation, congestion, or joint stiffness.

3. **Stay Informed**: Educate yourself about your health issue, including its causes, symptoms, and treatment options.

Stay up-to-date on pertinent research, treatment choices, and self-care behaviors advocated by healthcare experts.

4. **Develop Coping methods:** Build a toolbox of coping methods to assist you handle stress, worry, and emotional discomfort, which may lead to symptom flare-ups.

Practice relaxation methods, mindfulness meditation, deep breathing exercises, and guided imagery to increase tranquility and resilience.

5. **Implement Lifestyle Modifications:** Adopt healthy lifestyle practices that improve general well-being and lower the chance of symptom flare-ups.

Prioritize appropriate sleep, regular physical exercise, balanced diet, hydration, and stress management to enhance your body's capacity to deal with triggers and stresses.

6. **Maintain drug Adherence**: Follow your recommended treatment plan and drug regimen as instructed by your healthcare practitioner.

Take drugs regularly and stick to specified doses, timings, and precautions to control symptoms successfully and avoid flare-ups.

*7. **Create an Emergency Plan***: Develop a complete emergency plan describing procedures to follow in the case of a serious reaction or medical emergency.

Carry emergency drugs, such as epinephrine auto-injectors for severe allergies, and ensure that family members, caregivers, and colleagues are informed of your emergency action plan.

*8. **Seek Support:*** Reach out to friends, family members, support groups, or online communities for emotional support, encouragement, and practical guidance.

Connect with healthcare experts, including primary care doctors, specialists, therapists, and registered dietitians, who may give tailored advice and treatment alternatives.

*9. **Practice self-compassion***: Be kind to yourself and understand that treating chronic health issues entails ups and downs.

Practice self-compassion, patience, and resilience as you face the obstacles of living with flare-ups and responses.

*10. **Monitor Progress and Adjustments:***

Track your symptoms, treatment results, and lifestyle adjustments over time to assess progress and discover areas for improvement.

Be open to making revisions to your management plan depending on your growing requirements, preferences, and input from healthcare professionals.

Working with Healthcare Professionals

Working collaboratively with healthcare professionals is essential for effectively managing health conditions, addressing concerns, and optimizing overall well-being. Here are some key strategies for fostering positive and productive relationships with healthcare providers:

1. Open Communication:

- Maintain open and honest communication with your healthcare providers, sharing relevant information about your medical history, symptoms, concerns, and treatment preferences.

- Be proactive in asking questions, seeking clarification, and expressing any uncertainties or anxieties about your health condition or treatment plan.

2. Active Participation:

- Take an active role in your healthcare by actively participating in discussions, decision-making processes, and treatment planning with your healthcare team.

- Advocate for your needs, preferences, and goals, and collaborate with healthcare providers to develop personalized care plans tailored to your individual circumstances.

3. Ask Questions:

- Don't hesitate to ask questions about your diagnosis, treatment options, potential side effects, and long-term outcomes.

- Seek clarification on medical terminology, treatment protocols, and recommended lifestyle modifications to ensure a clear understanding of your healthcare plan.

4. Share Concerns and Feedback:

- Voice any concerns, challenges, or adverse reactions you may experience during treatment, and provide constructive feedback to your healthcare providers.

- Discuss any changes in symptoms, medication efficacy, or quality of life that may impact your overall health status and treatment goals.

5. Follow Treatment Recommendations:

- Adhere to your healthcare provider's recommendations, including medication regimens, dietary guidelines, lifestyle modifications, and follow-up appointments.

- Communicate any difficulties or barriers you encounter in adhering to treatment plans, and work collaboratively with your healthcare team to address them effectively.

6. Seek Second Opinions:

- Don't hesitate to seek second opinions or consult with specialists if you have unresolved medical concerns, complex health conditions, or treatment options that require further evaluation.

- Respectfully discuss your intention to seek additional input with your primary healthcare provider to ensure transparency and continuity of care.

7. Maintain Health Records:

- Keep organized records of your medical history, diagnostic tests, treatment plans, medication lists, and healthcare provider contact information.

- Provide updated health records to your healthcare team during appointments and consultations to facilitate comprehensive and coordinated care.

8. Attend Regular Check-Ups:

- Attend scheduled follow-up appointments, routine screenings, and preventive healthcare visits as recommended by your healthcare providers.

- Use these opportunities to discuss any changes in your health status, review treatment progress, and address emerging health concerns.

9. Be Respectful and Patient:

- Show respect, appreciation, and patience towards your healthcare providers, recognizing the complexity of their roles and the demands of their profession.

- Foster a collaborative and trusting relationship based on mutual respect, empathy, and a shared commitment to achieving your health and wellness goals.

10. Express Gratitude:

- Express gratitude and appreciation for the dedication, expertise, and compassionate care provided by your healthcare team.

- Acknowledge the positive impact of their efforts in supporting your health journey and improving your quality of life.

Chapter 7

Long-Term Maintenance and Prevention Strategies

Strategies for Preventing Histamine Build-Up

Preventing histamine build-up is crucial for individuals who experience histamine intolerance or sensitivity. By adopting specific dietary and lifestyle strategies, you can minimize histamine accumulation in the body and reduce the risk of histamine-related symptoms. Here are effective strategies for preventing histamine build-up:

1. Follow a Low-Histamine Diet:

- Limit consumption of foods high in histamine, including aged cheeses, cured meats, fermented foods (such as sauerkraut and kimchi), smoked fish, and alcoholic beverages (especially wine and beer).

- Choose fresh, unprocessed foods and prioritize cooking meals at home using fresh ingredients to minimize histamine exposure.

2. Identify and Avoid Trigger Foods:

- Keep a food diary to track your dietary intake and monitor for potential trigger foods that exacerbate histamine-related symptoms.

- Pay attention to individual food sensitivities and reactions, and gradually eliminate trigger foods from your diet to determine their impact on your symptoms.

3. Optimize Gut Health:

- Support a healthy balance of gut microbiota by consuming probiotic-rich foods such as yogurt, kefir, kombucha, and fermented vegetables.

- Incorporate prebiotic fiber sources like fruits, vegetables, whole grains, and legumes to nourish beneficial gut bacteria and promote digestive health.

4. Manage Stress Levels:

- Practice stress-reduction techniques such as mindfulness meditation, deep breathing exercises, yoga, or tai chi to mitigate the effects of stress on histamine levels and immune function.

- Prioritize self-care activities that promote relaxation and emotional well-being to reduce stress-related histamine release.

5. Stay Hydrated:

- Drink an adequate amount of water throughout the day to support hydration and detoxification processes in the body.

- Limit consumption of dehydrating beverages like caffeinated drinks and alcohol, which can exacerbate histamine-related symptoms.

6. Limit Histamine-Releasing Factors:

- Minimize exposure to environmental triggers that can stimulate histamine release, such as allergens, pollutants, chemical irritants, and extreme temperatures.

- Take precautions to avoid contact with known allergens and irritants, and create a clean and allergen-free environment in your home and workplace.

7. Consider DAO Enzyme Supplements:

- Discuss the potential benefits of diamine oxidase (DAO) enzyme supplements with your healthcare provider, especially if you have a deficiency in DAO production or impaired histamine metabolism.

- Take DAO supplements as directed before meals to help break down dietary histamine and support optimal digestion.

8. Practice Food Rotation:

- Rotate your dietary choices and vary your food selections to prevent overexposure to specific histamine-containing foods and minimize the risk of sensitization and intolerance.

- Incorporate a diverse range of fresh fruits, vegetables, proteins, and grains into your diet to ensure nutritional diversity and balance.

9. Monitor Medication Use:

- Be aware of medications that may exacerbate histamine-related symptoms or interfere with histamine metabolism, such as nonsteroidal anti-inflammatory drugs (NSAIDs) and certain antibiotics.

- Consult with your healthcare provider before starting or discontinuing any medications to assess their potential impact on histamine levels and overall health.

Gradual Reintroduction of Foods

Gradual reintroduction of foods is a structured approach used to identify food triggers, manage sensitivities, and expand dietary variety while minimizing the risk of adverse reactions. Here's how to implement gradual reintroduction effectively:

1. Start with Well-Tolerated Foods:

- Begin by reintroducing foods that are generally well-tolerated and have a lower likelihood of causing adverse reactions. These may include simple, minimally processed foods such as rice, chicken, certain vegetables, and fruits.

2. Introduce One Food at a Time:

- Introduce one food item at a time, preferably in its simplest form, without added seasonings or complex ingredients. This allows you to isolate the specific food and monitor your body's response accurately.

3. Monitor Symptoms:

- Keep a detailed food and symptom journal to track your dietary intake and any associated symptoms or reactions. Record the type and severity of symptoms, as well as the timing of their onset after consuming the reintroduced food.

4. Observe for Several Days:

- Allow sufficient time (usually 2-3 days) to observe for any delayed reactions or cumulative effects of the reintroduced food. Some reactions may not manifest immediately and can take time to develop.

5. Assess Tolerance Levels:

- Pay close attention to your body's response and assess your tolerance level to the reintroduced food. Note any changes in energy levels, digestion, mood, skin health, or other relevant indicators of well-being.

6. Gradually Increase Quantity and Complexity:

- If no adverse reactions occur, gradually increase the quantity and complexity of the reintroduced food over time. Experiment with different preparation methods, cooking techniques, and serving sizes to assess tolerance levels accurately.

7. Be Mindful of Potential Triggers:

- Exercise caution when reintroducing foods known to be common allergens or triggers for sensitivities, such as dairy, gluten, soy, nuts, eggs, and shellfish. These foods may require closer monitoring and slower reintroduction.

8. Consider Professional Guidance:

- Consult with a healthcare professional or registered dietitian experienced in food reintroduction protocols, especially if you have complex dietary restrictions, multiple food sensitivities, or underlying health conditions.

9. Listen to Your Body:

- Trust your body's signals and listen to its feedback throughout the reintroduction process. Honor any signs of discomfort, inflammation, or digestive distress by adjusting your dietary choices accordingly.

10. Practice Patience and Persistence:

- Understand that the process of reintroducing foods can be gradual and iterative. It may take time to identify individual tolerances, trigger foods, and optimal dietary patterns that support your health and well-being.

11. Stay Positive and Flexible:

- Approach food reintroduction with a positive mindset and a spirit of curiosity and experimentation. Embrace the opportunity to diversify your diet and explore new culinary experiences while remaining flexible and adaptive to your body's needs.

12. Celebrate Small Victories:

- Celebrate each successful reintroduction and milestone achieved along the way. Acknowledge your progress, resilience, and commitment to optimizing your dietary choices and overall health.

Frequently Asked Questions and Troubleshooting

Common Questions about the Anti-Histamine Diet

Here are some common questions about the anti-histamine diet along with their answers:

1. What is the Anti-Histamine Diet?

The anti-histamine diet is a dietary approach designed to minimize the intake of histamine-rich foods and reduce histamine levels in the body. It aims to alleviate symptoms associated with histamine intolerance or sensitivity, such as headaches, hives, digestive issues, and congestion.

2. What Foods Should I Avoid on the Anti-Histamine Diet?

Foods to avoid on the anti-histamine diet include aged cheeses, processed meats, fermented foods (e.g., sauerkraut, kimchi), alcoholic beverages, vinegar, smoked or cured fish, and certain food additives like sulfites and artificial preservatives. These foods are high in histamine or can trigger histamine release in the body.

3. Can I Eat Fresh Fruits and Vegetables on the Anti-Histamine Diet?

Yes, many fresh fruits and vegetables are considered safe on the anti-histamine diet. However, some individuals may be sensitive to certain fruits and vegetables due to their natural histamine content or ability to trigger histamine release. It's important to monitor your body's response and choose varieties that are well-tolerated.

4. Are There Any Supplements That Can Help with Histamine Intolerance?

Some individuals with histamine intolerance may benefit from supplements that support histamine metabolism or reduce allergic responses. These may include diamine oxidase (DAO) enzyme supplements, quercetin, vitamin C, and certain probiotics. However, it's essential to consult with a healthcare professional before starting any new supplements.

5. How Long Should I Follow the Anti-Histamine Diet?

The duration of the anti-histamine diet varies depending on individual needs, symptoms, and tolerance levels. Some people may follow the diet for a few weeks to identify triggers and alleviate acute symptoms, while others may choose to adopt it as a long-term lifestyle change. It's essential to listen to your body and make adjustments based on your unique health requirements.

6. Can I Eat Fermented Foods on the Anti-Histamine Diet?

Fermented foods are generally avoided on the anti-histamine diet because they can contain high levels of histamine and may exacerbate symptoms in individuals with histamine intolerance. However, some people may tolerate small amounts of fermented foods or choose varieties that are lower in histamine, such as fresh yogurt or kefir made from pasteurized milk.

7. Is the Anti-Histamine Diet Suitable for Everyone?

The anti-histamine diet may benefit individuals with histamine intolerance or sensitivity, but it may not be suitable for everyone. Pregnant or breastfeeding women, children, individuals with certain medical conditions, or those taking specific medications should consult with a healthcare professional before making significant dietary changes. Additionally, some people may not experience significant symptom relief with dietary modifications alone and may require additional medical evaluation and treatment.

8. Can I Reintroduce Foods After Following the Anti-Histamine Diet?

Yes, reintroducing foods after following the anti-histamine diet is possible, but it should be done gradually and with careful monitoring of symptoms. Pay attention to your body's response when reintroducing foods and identify any triggers or sensitivities that may contribute to histamine intolerance. It's essential to work with a healthcare professional or registered dietitian to develop a personalized reintroduction plan based on your individual needs and health goals.

9. What Are Some Common Symptoms of Histamine Intolerance?

Histamine intolerance can manifest in various symptoms, including headaches, migraines, nasal congestion, sneezing, itching, hives, flushing, digestive issues (such as bloating, gas, diarrhea, or constipation), fatigue, and anxiety. These symptoms can vary in severity and may occur shortly after consuming histamine-rich foods or beverages.

10. How Can I Identify Foods That Trigger Histamine Intolerance?

Keeping a detailed food and symptom journal can help identify patterns and pinpoint specific foods or ingredients that trigger histamine intolerance symptoms. Note the timing and severity of symptoms after consuming certain foods, as well as any other factors that may contribute to symptom flare-ups, such as stress, medications, or environmental triggers.

11. Can Cooking Methods Affect Histamine Levels in Foods?

Yes, certain cooking methods can impact histamine levels in foods. For example, high-temperature cooking methods like grilling, frying, or roasting may increase histamine levels in foods, while gentler cooking methods like steaming, boiling, or microwaving may help preserve lower histamine levels. Experiment with different cooking techniques to determine which ones are best tolerated.

12. Are There Any Support Groups or Resources for People with Histamine Intolerance?

Yes, there are various online forums, support groups, and resources available for individuals with histamine intolerance or sensitivity. These platforms provide opportunities to connect with others facing similar challenges, share experiences, exchange tips and recipes, and access valuable information and educational resources about managing histamine-related conditions.

13. Can Stress and Lifestyle Factors Impact Histamine Intolerance?

Yes, stress and lifestyle factors can influence histamine intolerance and exacerbate symptoms. Chronic stress, inadequate sleep, poor dietary choices, and environmental factors can all contribute to increased histamine levels and heightened sensitivity to histamine-rich foods. Practicing stress management techniques, prioritizing self-care, and adopting healthy lifestyle habits can help reduce histamine-related symptoms and improve overall well-being.

14. Is Histamine Intolerance the Same as Food Allergies or Sensitivities?

Histamine intolerance differs from food allergies or sensitivities in terms of underlying mechanisms and symptom presentation. While food allergies involve an immune response triggered by specific allergens, histamine intolerance results from impaired histamine metabolism or excessive histamine levels in the body. Histamine intolerance symptoms are typically non-immunological and may vary in severity and duration.

15. How Can I Ensure Nutritional Adequacy on the Anti-Histamine Diet?

Maintaining nutritional adequacy on the anti-histamine diet involves choosing a wide variety of nutrient-dense foods that provide essential vitamins, minerals, antioxidants, and macronutrients. Focus on incorporating nutrient-rich options like leafy greens, colorful vegetables, lean proteins, healthy fats, and whole grains into your meals to support overall health and well-being.

Addressing Challenges and Setbacks

1. Detect causes: Keep a comprehensive food and symptom log to detect trends and probable causes for histamine intolerance symptoms. This may help determine particular meals, environmental variables, or lifestyle practices that may worsen symptoms.

2. Plan and Prepare Meals: Plan your meals in advance and prepare histamine-friendly alternatives to ensure you have healthy and fulfilling choices easily accessible. Batch cooking, meal preparing, and stocking up on healthy products might make it simpler to keep to your nutritional plan.

3. Manage Social Situations: Communicate your dietary demands to friends, family members, and restaurant staff to ensure they understand your limits and can accommodate your choices. Offer to provide a food or propose histamine-friendly restaurant alternatives to make social events more pleasurable.

4. Seek Support and Guidance: Connect with support groups, online forums, or healthcare specialists that specialize in histamine intolerance for guidance, encouragement, and practical recommendations on managing your disease.

Consider working with a certified dietitian trained in histamine intolerance to design a tailored meal plan and address particular dietary difficulties.

5. Practice Self-Care: Prioritize self-care techniques that promote relaxation, stress reduction, and emotional well-being. Engage in activities such as meditation, yoga, deep breathing exercises, or hobbies that assist reduce stress and improve overall wellness.

6. Be Flexible and Adaptive: Understand that setbacks and struggles are a normal part of the road towards greater health. Be flexible and adaptable in your approach, and don't be too harsh on yourself if you meet roadblocks along the way.

7. Experiment and Adjust: Be open to experimenting with new meals, cooking techniques, and lifestyle tactics to discover what works best for you. Keep track of your progress and change your strategy depending on your specific requirements and preferences.

8. Focus on Progress, Not Perfection: Celebrate tiny successes and progress towards your health objectives, even if it's only making one beneficial adjustment at a time. Remember that consistency and tenacity are crucial to long-term success.

9. Stay updated and Educated: Stay updated on the newest research, resources, and advances relating to histamine intolerance and the anti-histamine diet. Knowledge helps you to make educated choices and advocate for your health successfully.

10. Listen to Your Body: Pay attention to your body's signals and recognise its demands and limits. Trust your instincts and intuition when it comes to choosing nutritional and lifestyle decisions that enhance your well-being.

Real-Life Success Stories and Testimonials

My journey with histamine intolerance began several years ago when I started experiencing unexplained symptoms like headaches, digestive issues, and skin rashes. Despite numerous doctor visits and medical tests, I struggled to find relief and answers to my persistent health problems.

It wasn't until I stumbled upon information about histamine intolerance that everything started to make sense. I learned that histamine-rich foods and environmental triggers were likely contributing to my symptoms and making me feel miserable.

Determined to take control of my health, I decided to embark on the anti-histamine diet journey. It wasn't easy at first, as I had to navigate through food restrictions and adjust to a new way of eating. However, with perseverance and commitment, I started to notice significant improvements in my overall well-being.

By eliminating high-histamine foods like aged cheeses, processed meats, and fermented foods from my diet, I experienced fewer headaches, less bloating, and clearer skin. I also incorporated more fresh fruits, vegetables, and lean proteins into my meals, which helped me feel more energized and nourished.

One of the most challenging aspects of managing histamine intolerance was dealing with social situations and dining out. However, with the support of understanding friends and family, as well as careful planning and communication, I was able to navigate social gatherings and enjoy meals without compromising my dietary restrictions.

Over time, I became more knowledgeable about histamine intolerance and how to manage it effectively. I learned to listen to my body, prioritize self-care, and make informed choices that supported my health and well-being.

Today, I'm happy to say that I've overcome many of the challenges associated with histamine intolerance, thanks to the anti-histamine diet and lifestyle changes. While I still have occasional flare-ups and setbacks, I feel empowered knowing that I have the tools and knowledge to manage my condition and live life to the fullest.

If you're struggling with histamine intolerance, I encourage you to explore the anti-histamine diet and seek support from healthcare professionals and online communities. With dedication, patience, and perseverance, you can reclaim your health and thrive despite histamine intolerance.

Chapter 8

Conclusion: Embracing a Balanced and Healthy Life

In conclusion, embracing a balanced and healthy life is essential for individuals managing histamine intolerance or sensitivity. The journey towards optimal health involves adopting a holistic approach that encompasses dietary modifications, lifestyle adjustments, and self-care practices tailored to individual needs and preferences.

Through the anti-histamine diet, individuals can minimize exposure to histamine-rich foods, reduce symptoms, and improve overall well-being. By prioritizing fresh, whole foods, incorporating nutrient-dense options, and avoiding common triggers, individuals can support histamine metabolism and maintain histamine balance in the body.

sHowever, managing histamine intolerance goes beyond dietary changes alone. It requires attention to other factors such as stress management, sleep hygiene, physical activity, and environmental awareness. By addressing these aspects of health, individuals can enhance immune function, optimize gut health, and reduce inflammation, contributing to a healthier and more resilient body.

Embracing a balanced and healthy life also involves fostering a positive mindset, practicing self-compassion, and cultivating meaningful connections with others. It requires flexibility, adaptability, and a willingness to learn and grow along the way.

As individuals navigate the challenges and triumphs of managing histamine intolerance, it's important to remember that progress is a journey, not a destination. Each step taken towards greater health and well-being is a testament to resilience, determination, and self-care.

By embracing a balanced and healthy life, individuals with histamine intolerance can reclaim their vitality, improve their quality of life, and thrive despite the challenges they may face. With the support of healthcare professionals, community resources, and personal determination, individuals can embark on a journey towards lasting wellness and fulfillment.

In the end, embracing a balanced and healthy life is not just about managing a health condition—it's about living life to the fullest, nourishing the body, mind, and spirit, and embracing the beauty of each moment along the way.

Encouragement for Continued Progress

As you continue on your quest to manage histamine intolerance and enjoy a balanced and healthy life, it's vital to recognize and appreciate the progress you've made so far. Every one of the steps that you take toward improved health, regardless of how insignificant they may seem, is a demonstration of your power, perseverance, and dedication.

To help you on your journey towards continuing improvement, the following words of encouragement are sent to you:

❖ Taking a minute to recognize and rejoice in the progress you've made in controlling histamine intolerance is an important step in the process of celebrating your accomplishments. Whether it's adhering to your nutrition plan, increasing the number of self-care practices you incorporate into your routine, or overcoming a particular obstacle, every accomplishment is worthy of being celebrated.

❖ Remind yourself that treating histamine intolerance is a journey, not a goal and that you should have faith in your path. Having faith in your abilities to overcome problems and hurdles along the way is essential, and you should have faith in the process itself. You should maintain your concentration on your objectives and have faith in the efficacy of tenacity and resilience.

❖ Being Kind to Yourself: As you navigate the ups and downs of managing histamine intolerance, it is important to practice self-compassion and kindness towards yourself. It is not a problem to have failures and periods of frustration; what is important is how you react to these experiences. Treat yourself with the same love and empathy you would show to a friend facing comparable challenges.

❖ Strive to maintain a cheerful and optimistic attitude by cultivating a positive mindset and concentrating on the opportunities and possibilities that are still to come. Approach each day with optimism, curiosity, and a readiness to learn and improve. Keep your eyes on the bright future you're creating for yourself, and let that vision drive you forward.

❖ Seek Support and Connection: Don't hesitate to reach out for support from friends, family members, healthcare professionals, or online groups. Surround yourself with individuals who understand and encourage you on your journey. Share your experiences, thoughts, and challenges with others, and draw strength from the connections you build along the path.

❖ Practice Patience and tenacity: Remember that healing and improvement take time, patience, and tenacity. Be kind to yourself as you traverse the challenges of managing histamine intolerance. Stay devoted to your health goals, and trust that your efforts will yield favorable results over time.

❖ Stay Educated and Informed: Continue to educate yourself on histamine intolerance, dietary strategies, and holistic approaches to well-being. Stay updated about new research, resources, and treatment choices that may benefit you on your journey. Knowledge helps you to make educated decisions and advocate for your health effectively.

❖ Celebrate Every Step Forward: Celebrate every minor triumph and milestone you attain along the way. Whether it's trying a new histamine-friendly meal, adopting a new self-care practice into your routine, or simply feeling better than you did yesterday, notice and honor your progress with appreciation and delight.

Above all, remember that your health and well-being are worth prioritizing. Embrace self-care, cultivate positivity, and nurture your body, mind, and spirit with kindness and compassion.

As you continue to move forward, may you find joy in the small moments, peace in the present, and hope for the future. Your journey towards wellness is a testament to your resilience and determination, and I believe in your ability to create a life filled with health, happiness, and fulfillment.

Wishing you strength, healing, and abundant blessings on your path ahead. You've got this!

9 798888 342788 5